BETRAYAL OF MINDS

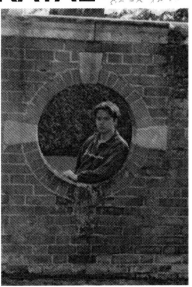

By Josephine Brown

'One million people commit suicide every year'
The World Health Organization

BETRAYAL OF MINDS

Published by
Chipmunkapublishing
PO Box 6872
Brentwood
Essex CM13 1ZT
United Kingdom

http://www.chipmunkapublishing.com

Edited by Mary Dow

Josephine Brown

CONTENTS

Introduction
Chapter 1   The Early Years
Chapter 2   Every Mother's Nightmare
Chapter 3   Traumatic Events
Chapter 4 Betrayal of Minds
Chapter 5   A Battle to be Fought
Chapter 6 The Tribunal Hearing
Chapter 7 Lack of GP Care
Helpful Information
Comments from the Author

BETRAYAL OF MINDS

INTRODUCTION

This is a journey through the Mental Health system, where I've stood many times in defence of my son David, aged just 13 years old. Such defence and absolute defiance is needed by a mother! I lost everything: my home, my marriage and, ultimately, my health. Was it worth it? Yes, it was. My reward – my son.

However, this book is intended to prevent the mentally ill and their relatives going through the same traumas as I had. The pitfalls have been many and the heartbreak considerable, but with each step in defiance I took, there was progress as a result.

Although progress was made, and this can only create changes, these changes are so badly needed within the Mental Health Services – you're invited to judge for yourself.

I dedicate this book to all the mentally ill and their carers, and hope beyond hope that life will become less hostile, and that the ignorance of others will eventually die, and the birth of 'compassion and understanding' will at long last prevail.

God Bless – Josephine

BETRAYAL OF MINDS

Josephine Brown

1. THE EARLY YEARS

I arrived at the hospital about to give birth, and in extreme pain. After tests were done, it became clear that the cord was around the baby's neck and the placenta was about to perforate. An emergency Caesarean section had to be performed. During the last moment that I remember before the surgery, I heard the surgeon referring to me as a 'poor cow'. I really wanted to reply to him, but was overcome by the anaesthetic. I haemorrhaged during the operation and lost three pints of blood.

My baby was born nearly dead and had to be resuscitated. When I awoke, I had no baby and looked like the evil dead. I'd been given a blood transfusion, but still had a bottle of blood attached to me. The doctors gave me a photograph of my baby and said that he'd been transferred by air ambulance to another hospital shortly after delivery. Three days later, I was transferred too, to be with him.

Trying very hard to hang on to my feelings, I shouted: 'Is there a vicar about?'
'No' came the answer.
I set off with my bottle of transfusion blood to find anyone who remotely resembled a man of the cloth. Yes, I found one, but he wasn't of my faith – he was Catholic. With the help of the staff gathered in the Special Care Baby Unit, my son was baptised into the Catholic faith and we named

BETRAYAL OF MINDS

him David.

My problems began in early pregnancy, when I received the blood test results of a woman who had a similar name to me. She received my test results confirming her unborn child was normal. I, on the other hand, received her test results confirming my unborn child would have spina bifida. Four doctors told me that I should have an abortion – but I refused. Instead, I asked for proof. But I didn't consider myself at the time to be a particularly brave person – and I wished that perhaps I'd kept my mouth shut.

I came face to face with the test known as an amniocentesis. The test was, to say the very least, absolutely awful. I'd been informed that the test could make me go into early labour. I could well believe this, because the shock experienced at having a huge needle about to pierce through one's bump and into the foetus is stuff that nightmares are made of. Playing for time – I remember asking the doctor to shut the window which had been left wide open.

I said nervously: 'Can you shut the window please? If things go wrong, I could descend through it!'

He then plunged the longest needle I'd ever seen into my vitals. I'd been given no anaesthetic, and I really wanted to change my mind about having this test done.

Josephine Brown

When he asked me if I wanted to watch, I believed him to be a sadist. I had this test performed in the early 70s and it isn't like today's technology or, at least, I hope it isn't.

The test results proved negative, but I was also told I was having a boy. After the birth of David, I did meet the other mum, who'd received my test results and, very sadly, her little baby girl had died. I could have sued the hospital, but didn't as they'd done everything possible to save my life and David's.

Six months later, I took David home. The nursing staff said he'd now sleep through the night. They were wrong – I was feeding him on demand for at least 12 months.

One day, I went to get up out of the chair and my legs wouldn't work. A GP was called; he gave me an injection and sent me to bed. He told me I was physically and mentally exhausted. Going to bed and remaining there for some three days was, I remember, like being given a free holiday.

Some three years later, David was just about sleeping through the night. But one day, David's heart stopped. He went on to suffer with respiratory problems. He was deaf – I'd been informed he suffered with high frequency deafness. He suffered iron deficiency, and his first teeth fell out, due to the huge amount of antibiotics he'd been given after his birth, which was, I believe, because he was suffering from pneumonia.

David's heart stopped again when he was three. He also had a weak immune system. I remember taking him to see a consultant, and I fell asleep half way through the consultation. His reaction was to gently wake me up, whereupon I apologised unreservedly. He then suggested taking David into hospital for a few days so that I could catch up on some sleep.

'What a nice man', I thought.
One week later, I found out that David had kept the nurses busy all night: they told me he'd been a handful.

When David reached four years old he became ill again − so we sold our home and bought a cheaper one. We took David to Sri Lanka, in the hope his health would improve. Our GP seemed to think we'd made a wise decision. Whilst in Sri Lanka, we stayed with the Mayor and his family in a most beautiful place called Matra. We stayed with them for three months. One day during our stay, it had been broadcast that many Tamils were going to land at Matra. The Mayor and his family had already fled to the capital, Colombo. We'd decided to lock the doors and hope for the best. The next day, having been deserted by the Mayor and his family, we decided to head for Colombo, too. I suggested taking the quickest route and going by train. The train was very crowded, so we travelled by taxi instead. Upon reaching Colombo, we heard the train we would have travelled on had blown up! However, we managed to get a flight back to the UK and returned home. David's health had greatly improved, and at last he seemed to be on the mend.

Whilst we were waiting at a bus stop one morning, a woman drove past us. She stopped her car and reversed. She asked if I'd consider David to become a model. I said I'd think about it, and she left me her business card. I took David for an interview and he was selected to model for TWA and Pan American Airways. His face was on billboards across the U.S. I was very proud of him.

When David was seven years old, his father died. I then took David and his sister Jane, who was ten, to Spain. We remained in Spain for three years. I worked for lawyers in Gibraltar, and life for us remained very positive. I returned to the UK and both children went to local schools in Hertfordshire. In 1991, I married Michael, whom I'd known since I was 18.

2. EVERY MOTHER'S NIGHTMARE

In 1993, we began experiencing problems with David, who was now at secondary school. He'd come home from school late. His behaviour was 'out of character'. He seemed very agitated. Trying to hold down a job and being worried sick about David's behaviour, I made a visit to his school, only to find he'd been suspended for smoking. I confronted David. He explained there was a boy at school selling cannabis – he'd been able to get it from the local ice cream van that stopped regularly at the school. Back to the school I went – saw the headmaster, said what I had to say. The head promised to look into matters immediately.

A few weeks passed. One day, when I was on my way home from work, I noticed the traffic was unusually heavy. I saw an ambulance and noticed a lot of people gathering. The ambulance wasn't ahead of me; it was down a verge leading off the main road, so I couldn't see much. I was just approaching my front door, when I heard the phone ringing. It was the local general hospital, who informed me that David had been involved in an accident and knocked down. I'd actually driven past my own son's accident. I reached the hospital – David only had a few cuts and bruises, which amazed me, because he'd been hit head-on and had been flung into the air, and had landed on the pavement.

Josephine Brown

David said to me, 'At least I was hit by a Toyota, Mum, not a Skoda'.
'What were you doing out of school?' I asked.
He replied: 'I went to see my girlfriend. But Mum, my dad saved me, because when I was flying in the air, he caught me and laid me gently down.'

I felt it best to listen, but not to comment, particularly as David's father had died when David was seven years old.

A few months later, David's behaviour became even more peculiar. He'd become aggressive, and, despite having the latest fashion clothes, he looked a complete mess. Adolescence was responsible for this, I thought. Meanwhile, my niece, Suzanne, visited us from the North of England.

She offered to give David a week's holiday. I agreed − but said to her that David must not come into contact with any alcohol or drugs. She, in turn, agreed to that. So I felt content that David would have a break and so would I, and off they all went. One week later, I received a phone call from Suzanne asking me for money − £60.00. I sent the money off.

The following week, I received a phone call from my sister, saying that Suzanne and her partner Jason had been giving David drugs. Mike and I couldn't get down the motorway fast enough!

BETRAYAL OF MINDS

On arrival at Suzanne and Jason's home. We hammered at the door. Suzanne asked me for more money! She told me that David had eaten a lot, and borrowed library books and not returned them. I didn't confront Suzanne at this point − my priority was to get David home. He looked terrible. He seemed very confused and very pale.

On the way home, David told me how Jason and Suzanne, had given him cannabis and opiates, and how David had saved Suzanne's baby's life by taking him upstairs out of the way of the thick black smoke of cannabis. The money they'd asked me for was supporting their habit. Needless to say, I was very angry, and I've not spoken to Suzanne since then.

I'm a firm believer in what goes around, comes around. To this very day, both Suzanne and Jason traffic drugs − but no action has ever been taken by the police, to my knowledge.

After a few weeks, David's behaviour was worse − he was now seeing things. He would say to me that he'd like me to meet John. I was happy to meet John, until I realised that John was invisible. He was a man whom David said kept going in and out of his bedroom. A further month or so passed, and David said he wanted to introduce me to his friends Elvis, Brenda and Shane. I was so relieved when Elvis, Brenda and Shane turned out to be real little people, and that I wasn't having to say hello to figments of David's imagination.

Two months later, David became worse. He'd lost weight, and was saying that we were trying to poison him. He believed his mother had died and I was a 'replica'. One evening, I was just about to eat, when David said to me: 'You're not my mother – I'm going to hit you'. He was holding a small hammer at the time.

I calmly replied: 'Well, if you're going to do that, do you mind if I eat my dinner first, as I can't go anywhere on an empty stomach!' He put the hammer down and came back to reality – just in time. Enough was enough. I phoned Social Services and explained that I needed help with my son. I was asked by a Mr Stevens where I worked. I said I worked for a firm of solicitors.

Mr Stevens then said: 'We don't normally deal with middle class people'. I explained that I was working class, purely because I went to work every day, like most people. Mr Stevens told me to send him on a 'young person's package holiday'.

'That should sort him out', he said.

I had no intentions of sending David away out of my sight ever again. David was now very ill indeed. He'd stopped eating altogether. I wanted so much to hug him as he lay motionless on his bed, but I couldn't because he didn't see me as his mother – just some 'replica'. For the next three days we went without sleep and became exhausted, as we'd had to restrain David from leaving the house. Again, feeling desperate, I contacted Social Services. This time, two social workers came along: a young woman called Linda and her colleague, Mike. I didn't know it at the time, but we were under investigation by them to see if David's condition had been caused by us.

Linda and Mike suggested that David be placed in hospital. Along came the GP and a hospital administrator, who was called Janet. All parties agreed that David should go to hospital. The GP phoned for an ambulance, which seemed to take forever to arrive. David, by this time, had grown very nervous and agitated. When it did arrive, Janet suggested that a blanket be placed over David's head. 'No, not whilst I'm his mum you won't. What planet are you from?' I said to her. 'The one called "Draconia"?'

I helped David into the ambulance and he was admitted to an adult psychiatric ward. The alternative was a drug abuse unit somewhere in Cambridge. I objected strongly when the word 'drugs' was mentioned − I didn't want David to be placed ever again anywhere near drugs. He was just 13 years old, very ill and very frightened.

Mike was a great support to both David and myself, which really helped. We'd not long been married, and now we were being driven to our very limits. Everything seemed to be crumbling. I remained at work, because we had a mortgage to pay. Even so, I visited David every evening. The doctors diagnosed David as suffering from paranoid schizophrenia. I didn't believe them for one moment.

I said: 'It's his ears and it's because he got knocked down'. It took me one whole year to accept that David had this terrible illness. One evening, I wrote this poem. It signalled the end of David's childhood and the beginning of a nightmare:

DAVID
He gazed into my eyes and I felt so humble,
My son, against all the odds, made me promise never again to grumble.
David is his name – a more courageous little guy
You could ever wish to meet
He forgives in an instance any bad comments made –
This young man is extremely brave.
Against medical opinions he fought for life and won –
Until, that is, schizophrenia had begun.

My son is my son, and yet I've lost part of him –
Now a new path we have to begin.
Injections once a week and pills every day –
Nothing, but nothing, can take this dreadful illness away.

BETRAYAL OF MINDS

A torment of mind, a torment of heart –
Will my son win his fight, or will his life depart?
What is this hell we're being put through?
What can I, as his mother, really do?

I watch the torment of his mind each day,
At night, I simply look at the stars in the sky and pray.
 I pray that his suffering and torment, which is very real
That someday his mind will somehow heal.

I pray to God to take away my pain
And let me have my son back once again.
I thank the doctors who once saved his life –
But he is now paying an enormous price.

I have my son in a physical sense –
But his eyes are vacant and his speech is spent.
His tortured mind is threatened so –
The ambulance is waiting – its time to go.

I shed the tears any mother would shed,
As my son is now tucked up in a hospital bed.
He thinks he is being punished for something he's done wrong –
How do I tell him schizophrenia has begun?

I love my son and want him to live
What quality of life, though, can this world give?
With bland remarks and hurtful eyes,
My son is in a world with little understanding and disguise.

Josephine Brown

Who would, given the choice,
Listen to the mentally ill so they have a voice?
To stand up for their views so that life can be
tolerable −
Very often they're accused of deeds quite horrible:

If one has killed, the rest are the same −
This world accuses them all − is the system to
blame?
I've met some fabulous people who are mentally ill
− their expectations of life are small; they fight for
normality in their lives − this is all.

Cannot we, as a nation, give the mentally ill love,
care and support?
Or do we, when something terrible happens,
simply say it's someone else's fault?

Whilst on this ward, David tried to take his life, but
the ward staff didn't inform me. He cut his wrists. I
found out by visiting him, and was very angry. I
asked for an explanation from the ward sister.

She said: 'We don't have to inform relatives; there
is no legal requirement for us to do so'.
I replied: 'Well, you're wrong − my son is still only
13 years old, and considered a minor. Therefore I
should have been informed.'

I enlisted the help of a local solicitor − just to be
told by him: 'Well, if you have a son like that,

you're always going to be in trouble with him!'

Thanks for nothing, I thought, and left.

One afternoon, David had managed, I don't quite know how, to phone and speak to the Lord Chancellor's office in London. He told them he'd been kidnapped and held against his will in hospital. Within 20 minutes, police arrived to investigate. This time, however, staff informed me. I'd always told David that if he ever felt he was in a dangerous situation to phone for help wherever possible. This advice he obviously remembered.

After a few months, David was allowed home; he needed weekly maintenance injections. I watched as his little body shook with the side-effects. His mental outlook was not good: obviously, he was still very confused and, to be honest, he displayed immense courage even though he was still very ill. It's difficult enough to come to terms with any illness as an adult – but now, here was a frail 13 year-old boy, completely unaware of the seriousness of his illness, but having to deal with the consequences of it.

He'd become frightened of cars – particularly the headlights. He saw life very differently to us. Mike and I were filled with a mixture of fear and insecurity for the future, anger, hopelessness of the situation; but, still, compassion. We couldn't tell anyone, especially our work colleagues – the stigma of David's illness was just too great.

We were still trying to hold down our jobs and keep everything together. Jane was about to leave secondary school. She'd found herself a boyfriend. We all soldiered on the best way we could. When David was out of hospital, I took my holiday entitlement to care for him. Mike and I took it in turns to care for David. We attended a hospital Outpatient check up with David – the doctors decided to change his medication to a less effective drug. The effects on David were awful. His illness came back with a vengeance. I asked his GP to call and assess David's mental state and to request that David be put back on the drug he'd been used to.

David's GP couldn't attend, but sent another in his place. This GP, I knew – he'd been a doctor at the hospital. He'd obviously applied to become a doctor in general practice. This GP was, to say the least, rude and obstructive, and, above all, wasn't listening to us. I asked him to leave, as he was obviously unable to assist us, and we really didn't need his lack of courtesy at a time when we needed support. I requested David's GP to call when he could.

Time was ticking on: another day of trying to cope with David's illness. Until, finally, David slipped out of the house and ran into trouble with the law. David was arrested and when I arrived at the police station, I asked the duty officer that David be placed back in hospital.

BETRAYAL OF MINDS

The alternative was a young offenders' detention centre. David's psychiatrist arrived at the police station, and David was then returned to the psychiatric unit.

A few days later, David was placed under Section 3 of the Mental Health Act. Again, without my knowledge: David's GP and two hospital doctors placed David under the Section. This, again, was wrong. I should have been present, or, at the very least, kept informed. I experienced difficulties with the staff on the ward. I'd made friends with the other patients on the ward. I helped them by going to the Post Office to cash their money. I also helped them with their benefit entitlements, and they called me 'the Angel of Welwyn Ward'. I was quite flattered − but felt I'd only done what anyone else would have done (how naïve I was).

I had, without realising it, made myself unpopular with the staff. I was told not to help the patients. I was also told that I wouldn't be able to visit David as often as I did. Tough, I thought. In fact, I'd have to make sure I spent more time with David, provided my visits were within the permitted hospital visiting hours.

There was absolutely nothing they could do about it. From 2 pm until 9 pm daily, I sat keeping David and other patients company, with a certain air of quiet self-assured defiance. No one challenged me today, I thought − but tomorrow may be different.   .

After a few days on the ward, David refused to take his medication.   His mental state wasn't good.   What happened next didn't warrant the heavy handedness that occurred. Two nursing assistants came running towards David and myself. David was at this time a frail, very frightened young man, and I'm slim and under 5ft. So when you have two large nursing assistants stampeding towards you, you may well think like I did: that they'd hopefully stampede past you. They didn't.

Instead, they dragged poor David to the ground. They yelled at me to leave. I didn't leave.   I watched in sheer horror as one of the nursing staff injected David. By this time, David was screaming for me.   He yelled and screamed several times, then it went very quiet.   They'd literally dragged David into a side room.

I said to them: 'There was no need for this − I could have got David to take his medicine.'

 I went into the room − David was lying very still.

In fact, I thought they'd killed him. Tears were rolling down my face, and I knew then that if this was how David was going to be treated, and the total lack of regard that was shown for myself as David's mother − that we were both in for a difficult time.   I then decided to write down everything that occurred on this ward.

Due to the shock of witnessing David being dragged off and the hopelessness of the situation, I knew I'd have to become stronger emotionally. It was on that very day I changed. I thought if this was the way life on this ward was going to be, then I'd have to let them find out just what I was made of!

3. TRAUMATIC EVENTS

When I visited David, I found the staff difficult in their attitude towards him. On this ward you got used to seeing and hearing things you'd rather not have witnessed. You also got used to being told about the rules that you must follow − but the staff appeared to be exempt. In particular, nurses would sneak into the patients' smoking room and puff away − but when visitors attempted to do this, they were told not to. I raised a complaint, and a sign was erected on the door.

A ward sister said to me that she 'had a bone to pick with me'. She yelled from one end of the ward to the other.

I went into her room and sarcastically said to her: 'If you're upset about something, perhaps you should see the on-call doctor.'

She replied: 'Why have you prevented David from having the appropriate medication?'

I presume she was referring to David's psychiatric consultant wishing for my consent for David, aged now just 14, to be placed on the drug clozapine. This drug I had watched half kill another patient. I'd done my homework on this drug, and the side-effects could certainly kill David. Apparently, this particular drug is so dangerous that it has to be monitored on a monthly basis: patients have to give regular blood samples and have to become registered in order to take it.   It can cause a condition called neutropenia, in which there is a fall in the number of white blood cells (neutrophils).

When this happens, the body is less able to resist infections, and this can, albeit rarely, be fatal. David had to be given high doses of antibiotics when he was born. Prolonged use destroyed David's teeth and wiped out his immune system. Bearing all this in mind, I felt this drug wasn't for David, at least not yet. No other antipsychotic drugs should be administered as well as clozapine.

Back to the sister's comments.

I said to her: 'I've never stopped David having Depixol (an anti-psychotic maintenance drug).' Even on this drug, I've watched David shake uncontrollably. He'd be given another drug to combat this, called procylidine. All of these drugs were difficult enough to come to terms with, but clozapine, I had no doubt, could be fatal for David.

'Don't you want your son to get better?' she said.

'Of course I do, but I'll not consent to a drug that could bring about David's death.'

One afternoon, I received a surprise visit from a social worker, Jean, who called at my home.

Josephine Brown

She was quite blunt. She said: 'I suppose you know – if you don't consent to David having clozapine, he'll end up spending the rest of his life locked away.'

I replied: 'You appear to be blackmailing me.'

Jean remained quiet. She just happened to have a consent form handy. She handed it to me.
I ripped it up and said to her: 'Please close the door on your way out. I can't and won't be blackmailed by you or anyone else. If you lock David away for the rest of his life then I will have to spend the rest of my life fighting to set him free.'

Jean left – I never ever saw her again. I believe she moved home, possibly to retire.

Little did she know that after she'd left my house that day I'd shed many tears. It seemed that I had little choice but to consent to the use of clozapine, and did so by sending a letter to David's consultant, whereupon David was given this drug.

I continued to spend every day on the ward. The staff thought I was irritating them deliberately, but I was there to support David. If that upset the staff, then it was their problem.

David's confidence had deteriorated. He'd spend many hours not talking to me. I thought I'd give David something to look forward to. I said to him: 'What if I can get you out for the weekend?'

BETRAYAL OF MINDS

He replied: 'This weekend?'

I said: 'Why not? I could try.'

I asked for David to come home for the weekend, but this was turned down. However, I was told I could take him out for a few hours. I couldn't wait to tell David. We'd got five hours, and we headed home on the bus.

I mentioned earlier that David had shown courage throughout his illness − when it was time to return to the hospital, he didn't complain, although I knew if it had been me I wouldn't have wanted to return. It was only when we reached the lift to the ward that he hesitated.

I said to him: 'We can always go out again and I'll stay with you for a while − OK?'

As time went by, David and I had many trips out. His illness was unresponsive to the maintenance drugs. It was in April 1994 I consented to the drug "Clozapine". When I was attending a ward round, a nursing assistant came up to me and informed me that David's psychiatrist had gone to America to study the use of 'mixing drugs'. That explained his absence − it's normal for the consultant psychiatrist to be in attendance.

I never really took a lot of notice until the

unforgivable happened. Whilst visiting David one evening, I'd noticed he was very pale. This in the past had always served as a warning that David would become unwell physically. Apparently, that evening, David had been administered clozapine, Depixol, two diazepam tablets, two paracetamol tablets for a toothache, and procylidine. I believe the use of other drugs with clozapine is not recommended. I told the staff several times that David didn't look well, but they didn't listen to me. My gut feelings told me that something was wrong, but I didn't know what.

I left the ward that evening at 9 pm.

Next day, I arrived on the ward and went into David's bay – he wasn't there. I asked another patient if he'd seen David.

'Don't you know?' he said.

It was at that moment I was glad I'd not eaten any breakfast.

I asked: 'Well, where is he?'

The patient explained that about 11 pm – some two hours after I'd left the hospital – the crash team had come up from A & E to resuscitate David as his heart had given out. Feeling very angry, but at the same time trying to control my anger, I went in search of a member of staff. I spoke to the ward sister and simply asked why I hadn't been informed of what could have been my son's last moments on this earth.

She replied: 'We're under no legal obligation to inform you.'

'But I'm his mother and he's still under 16.'

I then said to her: 'If David had been a patient on a general medical ward, staff would have informed me of his condition. Why and how could this situation been allowed to occur, just because David is a mental health patient?'

An abuse of both my rights and David's had occurred.

'So, where is he?' I asked the sister. 'Well, he had to be taken into a side ward – third on the left.'

I nearly cried when I saw poor David – he was well out of it. I sat by his bedside, my hands holding my face. My anger had turned into a state of sheer hopelessness. I felt like carrying David off somewhere safe.

I now believed David's life to be compromised. I believed, that night David had been the subject of 'polypharmacy'. This is the name given to the dubious practice of prescribing a cocktail of drugs at the same time, thereby increasing the risks of adverse effects. This can diminish a person's quality of life, and, occasionally, it can be life-threatening. I wrote complaint after complaint to the Mental Health Act Commission about the way David and I had been treated.

All kinds of things were wrong about this ward. For instance, the patients had no means of drying their clothes. I purchased a tumble dryer and had it delivered to the ward. Thefts were commonplace amongst the staff – patients' cigarettes would go missing. Two elderly sisters systematically took the patients' sandwiches home. Once, I watched an elderly nursing assistant throw a patient to the ground. An older gentleman spent precisely one week on the ward. He was given his medication one night – he was dead in the morning.

 A nurse was later seen crying; she was then transferred to another ward. Worst of all, David witnessed a young man taking his own life – drowning whilst in the bath.

Staff could be incredibly cruel. For instance, they'd give consent for David to come home with me. They'd watch him become excited. I'd turn up to collect him and then they'd say he couldn't go. The boy cried himself to sleep many times. No-one is perfect – but, my God, how long must I bear witness to this abuse of very vulnerable people?

In March 1995, Mike and I were getting into financial difficulties – we were having problems paying the mortgage. Although I was still working, our mortgage repayments were nearly double what they had been. We'd tried to fight a notice to quit served on us by the Building Society. The bailiffs were at the front door – whilst Social Services let themselves in the patio doors. To make matters worse, we were reduced to three teabags to last nearly a week.

Jane had fallen pregnant and gave birth to a little girl.

On the same night that Jane went into hospital, Mike suffered a heart attack at 4 am.

I visited Jane in the maternity ward, Mike in coronary care and David in the psychiatric unit. Later, I sat in the grounds of the hospital, smoking a cigarette and wondering what the hell to do. I realized that I'd rushed out the house in such a hurry that I'd left my purse at home, which meant I had to walk home.

The hospital was two miles from where we lived, and normally I'd be hesitant to rush back – but after the evening we'd all had, I really never gave a thought to my own safety, although I should have done. Anyway, I reached home safe and sound, but very tired.

In the morning, I phoned the hospital to see how everyone was. I then phoned my boss, whose name was Alan. I explained to Alan what had happened. I then said that I'd not be in for the day.

To my amazement, he snapped at me: 'Well, Jo, I'm running a business and I really cannot do without you for the day – I've got a lot to do, so I'd appreciate it if you would come in, because I can't really guarantee your job if you don't.'

'OK,' I said, 'I'll be there at 10 am.'

I'd never had time off before. On one occasion, whilst ill at work with flu, even the senior partner expressed his concerns and told me to go home – but Alan refused to let me go. So I stood no chance of not going to work that morning. We needed the money, especially since our eviction was becoming inevitable.

Meanwhile, back on the ward, most patients, when they became difficult, were threatened by staff.

They would say: 'You'll be sent to Fairfield.'

Having listened to this threat many times, I asked one of the patients who'd been to Fairfield just exactly what it was all about.

'I quite like it,' said one patient. 'I much prefer it to being here.'

Staff would instil fear into the patients about this place. It was as though a form of torture went on there. The threats worked though – often difficult patients would cease their bad behaviour in order to remain where they were.

I never thought that I'd be visiting David at Fairfield. In a way, though, I'm glad I did, if only to see the place; although it was old and strict-looking, the resident psychiatrist and staff were lovely, compared to what David and I had been used to. However, David was sent there by mistake.

It transpired that a hard-of-hearing patient had been placed in the same bay as David. This guy had tried to hurt David. Staff saw red marks on David's throat and, later that day, David was sent to the blackened pits of Fairfield. When I met the Consultant Psychiatrist at Fairfield, he said he didn't quite know why David had been sent there. Anyhow, I explained that the staff where David had come from were trying to instill fear among the patients regarding Fairfield. I also said to him, defensively, that should anything happen to my son whilst he was in his care, then I would certainly take matters further.

The psychiatrist dispelled my apparent fears and took me on a tour around the wards. All the patients seemed well cared for and none had apparently lost their fingers, toes or hands by being placed there. The psychiatrist, a well-respected man, took a very dim view of the staff on Welwyn Ward. He said that they shouldn't threaten their patients in this way, and cause them distress.

David had been placed in Fairfield's care for approximately three weeks. After the first week, the doctor said that he didn't know why David had been sent to a 'locked ward'. Clearly, the boy's behaviour didn't require him to be on a secure ward. He, therefore, to my absolute delight, allowed David to come home with me for the remaining two weeks, before being sent back to his usual hospital. Whilst visiting Fairfield the next day to pick David up, I noticed the presence of the hard-of-hearing patient. I'd been informed the hospital had got it wrong, and had sent the wrong person – David, instead of the hard-of-hearing patient. This man obviously had severe learning difficulties on top of suffering a mental illness, and, furthermore, was severely hard of hearing. Wouldn't a little compassion or help have been more valuable to this man than, most likely, scaring him out of his wits by sending him to the dreaded Fairfield?

After two weeks of sheer delight at having my son at home, my happiness was destroyed once again. Whilst I was preparing a meal for David, the men in white coats arrived in an ambulance. I hadn't noticed as I was in the kitchen, oblivious to the knock on the door. They took David by his arms and bundled him into the ambulance and informed me they were taking him back to Welwyn Ward. There seemed little point in enquiring if he could have his dinner.

No, this wasn't to happen. After they'd taken David I was reduced to tears. I threw his dinner away and my daughter Jane, upon seeing the ambulance arrive, came rushing in and caught me crying. Not a sight I like my children to see, even if they are young adults. I was embarrassed beyond belief and, I believe, heartbroken. After a while, I decided to go to the hospital to 'pick up the pieces' for David. No-one had pre-warned me; I believe Welwyn Ward had found out that David had been at home and had decided to retrieve him.

Two weeks later, I was walking home when my son- in-law came running towards me, saying that David had been knocking at my front door. I hurried home, to find David in a very distressed state. We got inside the house and David told me he'd run away from the hospital, and could I hide him in the loft? Every difficult moment I've ever had with David has occasionally had its funny moments as well, and this was indeed one of them.

I said to David: 'I can't hide you in the loft because we don't have one.'

'How about the cellar?' he said.

Josephine Brown

'We haven't got one of those either!'

I told him to go to his bedroom, where I'd bring him a drink and we'd discuss what to do next. His shirt had been torn where he'd hidden in the bushes in the hospital grounds. He also began to have an asthma attack, but luckily I'd always kept a spare inhaler at home, so that proved useful.

After about an hour, I told David that, although I really didn't want to, I'd have to let the ward know where he was. At first he was mortified – but I told him this time I'd go there with him. He agreed, and after phoning the hospital, a police car arrived. David began telling the officers that he'd run away because the staff were horrible to him. We reached the hospital and approached the ward via the lift. To my astonishment, a member of staff began telling David off, whereupon the police officer said to her: 'If you weren't so horrible to him, he wouldn't have run away!'

Nice one, I thought – but I kept my applause for this remark completely under wraps. The officer then asked me if I'd like a lift back home. I told him that I'd take the bus, as I intended to stay with David for awhile. My remark immediately led to the nursing sister giving me a look of loathing. I thanked the officer and stayed with David until the end of visiting hours.

I remained on that ward day in and day out, until

the staff created difficult situations so that I would leave. They informed me that I must not visit David in his bay. Something I'd been doing for at least two years. I sent the ward manager a letter of complaint saying that I, like many other visitors, don't possess the gift of clairvoyance. Therefore, unless they erect a sign displaying their apparent new rules, then, legally, they cannot enforce them. The next day, wearing a most wicked smile, I proceeded to visit David in his bay. Two days later, upon entering his bay, I found a sign displaying the new rules. However, the sign was displayed inside the bay and not outside. I immediately called one of the nursing assistants, asking them to erect their new sign upon the outside. A few days passed, and upon paying and helping myself to a coffee, I was asked if I'd paid for my drink. Petty, irritating little situations like that were frequently created by the staff. I was requested yet again not to visit as often.

I replied: 'Sorry no can do.' Again, I raised complaint after complaint regarding the staff's treatment of their patients. I'd witnessed two deaths, and there were more deaths to come. I knew, at some stage, this ward and its staff would be held accountable. Indeed, a few years later, the hospital was found guilty of 'complacency' towards the patients in their care. Thereafter, life changed on this ward for the better. However, many lives had been lost in order to secure this change of policy and attitudes.

Before such changes occurred, and whilst David remained on the ward, University students were employed to watch and take notes on the patients. These people had no training and no idea how to react to difficult situations. I felt sorry for them and for the patients. I'd begun to look upon all the patients as potential victims; however, there were one or two members of staff who were dedicated and who genuinely helped patients, and to them I'm very grateful.

I realised David's illness was extremely unpopular with the staff – but I was being made to pay a high price, along with David, by them, merely because I loved my son. Another staff member, an Asian man who'd recently become employed on the ward, began making sexual gestures towards David. I challenged him about this and said I'd be taking matters further, to the police. He denied David's allegations, thinking, of course, that the mentally ill couldn't possibly be believed. I further asked him how long he'd been in the UK, and did he have any qualifications or right to stay and work in this country? This guy disappeared from the ward almost overnight.

Yes, I'd become a pain in the neck to the nursing staff and to the psychiatrist, whom I threatened with Injunction proceedings if he ever tried to have David removed to another establishment without my prior knowledge. I knew too that, because I spent all day with my son for every day of his life on this ward, I wasn't liked. I didn't care whether I was liked or not. In order to feel unhappy regarding the views of the ward staff, you have to firstly respect and like them. I clearly didn't respect or like these individuals. They were, after all, being paid to care for the mentally ill, but they often made life very difficult, if not impossible for their patients. Had I been able to trust, respect and generally feel comfortable with the staff's behaviour towards their patients, I wouldn't have remained so vigilantly every day in support of David. Possessive − no, protective − yes.

Another day, another incident. Staff were commencing their shift, and I was about to leave the ward. Mike was sitting down, and I got ready to leave, saying that I'd meet him downstairs. Some staff members entered the lift and decided to block my way into it − as though I was a patient trying to escape.

Everyone was laughing, including Mike.

David came up to me and said: 'Never mind, Mum, let them have their little joke.'

I was hurt that Mike had also found it amusing − I could hardly speak to him. I felt betrayed, and I had been.

After many months, David's psychiatrist held a meeting with one of his colleagues who was also a

Josephine Brown

Consultant psychiatrist, but at a private establishment. They'd apparently agreed that David would be transferred. However, they'd forgotten to let me know!

They didn't inform me of their decision, nor had I seen the new hospital. In fact, I visited David, thinking he was still at his usual hospital. It was then, and only then, that I learned that David had already travelled by ambulance to a hospital near Cambridge. I was informed that a nursing assistant had travelled with him. None of David's medical notes had gone with him to this hospital – so the doctors and nursing staff at this place wouldn't be aware of any of David's physical health problems and/or mental health records. These records, despite my repeatedly asking for them to be sent to the new hospital, were never sent and were, apparently, lost! How convenient, I thought. I telephoned the new hospital, and was told that David had been placed, yet again, on a locked ward.

This hospital was a private hospital. The fees at that time were £300.00 per day; this was funded by the taxpayer. I was unaware at the time that the local funding office had agreed that David should only remain at this hospital for a maximum of two years. Yet again, no letter had arrived at my home to inform me regarding David being transferred to this hospital, nor had it been discussed with me earlier. I even had to ask the admissions office for the address. I'd already obtained the telephone number from directory enquiries. No member of Social Services had contacted me, and I felt very much alone.

My home had been repossessed, my marriage seemed doomed and now my son had been taken to a place I knew nothing about. His future seemed out of my hands. But soon, I ceased feeling sorry for myself − I rang the hospital and I told them I'd be visiting David the next day. I didn't wait for them to say yes or no.

Mike and I visited David at this highly expensive hospital situated near Cambridge - namely Kneesworth House Hospital. I'd noticed along the way there were no buses and it was a fair way from the railway station. We drove into the huge grounds, went to the reception area and requested to see David. We had to sign in and were given a badge. We walked along the corridor, and at the far end was the ward. We rang the bell and were shown into the ward. We saw David − he looked very frightened, very confused and very resentful. He thought I'd placed him there, and I tried desperately to convince him I hadn't known anything about his being moved there. David explained that he'd spent a very long time in the ambulance and he was very scared. He hadn't known where he was going. The staff asked me if I could have his hospital notes sent to them as they didn't know what anti-psychotic drugs David had been administered.

Upon hearing this, I asked them how they intended to treat David, not knowing what drugs he'd been on at his previous hospital?

'It's up to the doctor,' the staff replied.

'This just gets better!' I thought.

'How long will David be staying?' I asked.

'Don't know, the hospital social worker will let you know.'

Mike and I tried to comfort David, but in my heart of hearts I knew where one battle had ceased, another was about to begin. I left that hospital quietly angry, but, more importantly, I felt so very sorry for David, and became determined that I would somehow secure his freedom. Out of this tragic situation came hope, and at least the staff seemed more humane in their approach towards their patients. I was feeling like I'd given birth to a baby and then had that child stolen, and I didn't know when or if it would be returned. I focused on how I could visit David, as this hospital was so far away. Mike and I managed four evenings a week and one visit at weekends. It was hard going, but I knew I had to be there for David. The hospital decided to stop any drugs that David may have been given by the previous hospital. Despite many requests for his notes, no notes were forthcoming. Due to the lack of medication, David tried to end his life. He was now on 24-hour watch

BETRAYAL OF MINDS

by staff. At least I'd been informed.

Such was David's mental state when I visited him on my own, that he said to me: 'Who are you?'

'I'm your mum,' I replied.

'I don't know you,' he said.

I left the ward for a few moments and then returned and said: 'Hi Dave'.

David looked at me. A few seconds passed. Then he said: 'Hello Mum'.

Kneesworth Hospital, had now after some time recommenced administering clozapine. I'd told them that this, along with the drug Depixol , had also been given to David whilst on Welwyn Ward at the QE11 hospital. They were not happy at hearing this.

On one of my visits, after only just a few days, David seemed dirty, scruffy and generally unwell. I told the staff that I wanted to see his doctor. I was given her telephone number, and I told her that I felt my son looked as though he'd been sleeping in a dustbin. I told her I wasn't happy, and I expected to see an improvement upon my next visit. After a short time, David was assaulted by another patient. He was punched in the face whilst eating his dinner.

When I commented about this, the staff apologised to me. On another occasion, David was assaulted yet again whilst he was on the telephone speaking to me. He was kicked in the lower back and punched in the face. This time, I lodged a complaint.

I began to fear for David's life. I told his psychiatrist that such attacks on David should not be occurring.

She replied: 'It's no more than what you should expect from this type of establishment.'

I told her that unless such attacks ceased, then I would be taking legal proceedings. I informed her that the hospital had a duty of care for David and they were lacking in that duty of care. Five more assaults upon David occurred over a period of three years. I employed a solicitor for David; although this solicitor presumably meant well, he wasn't a strong enough character to defend David against this lot. The mere fact that David attended the ensuing tribunal hearing was sufficient for both of David's psychiatrists. I made them aware that it was my intention to defend David against their Draconian views. After all, the taxpayers (including me) were paying a high price for David's care – the fees were now £400 per day.

BETRAYAL OF MINDS

David had endured a total of eight serious assaults. On one occasion, Mike and I travelled to the hospital in the early hours and found David bruised and battered. We informed the police. The hospital weren't going to, but we insisted. We also insisted they call the duty doctor to examine David. This duty doctor was, to say the least, a waste of space. He should have sent David to another hospital so that his injuries could be treated, but he didn't. We asked one of the administrators to take photographs of David's injuries. This he did, and gave them to us. After a short time, the police arrived and said that the staff of this hospital were going to have to 'get their act together'.

'There have been too many deaths here,' said the officer to us. The administrator of the hospital admitted that deaths had indeed occurred. A Tribunal Hearing was arranged. David's psychiatrist said to me that I'd be taken to the 'highest order' because I'd made allegations against them.

At the Tribunal Hearing they said that David wasn't well enough to be discharged. I challenged this as much as I could, but knew within my heart that this was true. However, my defence of David would continue. I left the hearing feeling very aggrieved that David may have to endure further assaults. I didn't know if or when such assaults would end David's life. I wrote further letters of complaint that this overrated, expensive hospital seriously lacked a duty of care towards my son.

I threatened more legal proceedings against them, although I was bluffing. I couldn't afford a solicitor to act for me. Our house had been repossessed and, shortly afterwards, Mike and I divorced. I made visits to see David by train and taxi. I was in no position to enter expensive litigation proceedings. But again, only I knew that – they didn't. I pressed on with further threats – David's consultant, in turn, passed on my letters to his legal team.

I had a breakthrough at last. The consultant's legal team agreed with me that there was a lack of duty of care. Suddenly, David was being transferred to a bungalow within the hospital grounds, with no locked doors. This would be a more tranquil place for David, and would give me a little more peace of mind, I thought.

I was still working and living on my own in a two bed roomed flat. One morning, when I was getting ready for work, I fell against the radiator; my right arm wouldn't work. My eyes were dull and glazed. After a few minutes, I managed to look again at myself in the mirror – I really had problems recognising myself.

I'd suffered a stroke, according to the neurologist – although by the time I got to see him, it was several months after this had occurred. I told him that there were worse cases than me, and that I was fine. He apologised to me for the delay, but insisted he examine me.

I told him that my vision had been impaired and my right arm had been paralysed at the time, but that I'd recovered after a short period of time.

'You've suffered a short stem ischaemic stroke.'

He explained to me that most stroke victims are unaware they've suffered a stroke and so deny it. I think it's a condition of the brain whereby it just doesn't register just what you've suffered. Stroke or no stroke − I still managed to visit David at the hospital. A few months later, I began feeling quite ill; I phoned my sister, thinking that she may visit me. I was very tearful and I could hardly breathe. She told me to either get an ambulance or go to bed. I felt that unwell that I chose to go to bed. To my complete astonishment, I woke up three days later.

I had got divorced from Mike some months earlier. It was my decision that once Mike had moved out of my life I'd live as independently as possible. I'd been granted a divorce on the grounds that my marriage to Mike had irretrievably broken down and I couldn't be expected to live with him. I'd tried to remain friends with him, but found his presence in my life, albeit helpful, was making me ill. I'd got over Mike's betrayal at the hospital, but couldn't get over him comparing me, on a daily basis, to a woman he knew where he worked. I didn't need that humiliation. At the same time of course, I was also aware that my continued defence of David's illness had possibly become too much for Mike. At least he was now free of any commitments towards me and my family. He moved out and I was left with my two-bedroomed council flat. It was a pretty place, even though I'd come to think of it as a 'sick flat' because I'd been so ill there. There were some aspects of my present life I did like − I felt safe there and my neighbours were great. But I was now living on Incapacity Benefit and Income Support. I didn't know how I'd be able to visit David as often as I did. Income Support would only allow for one visit a week. This didn't stop me writing complaints, though. Upon arriving on one of my visits, I said 'hello' to a hugely-built nursing assistant.

Then I said: 'There's no sugar', as I began helping myself to a cup of tea.

The assistant replied: 'You can always write a letter of complaint about it.'

Instead of taking offence, I was quietly pleased that I was managing to acquire a reputation. The next time I visited David and went to help myself to my usual drink, a notice had been displayed which said 'No visitors allowed into the staff area'. I'm really getting to them, I thought, which is nothing compared to what this hospital has put me through over the years.

After about eight months living in the hospital bungalow, David designed a Christmas card. I was informed he'd won an award called the Koestler Award. I hadn't a clue what this award was, but I was hugely proud of David. His Christmas card was exhibited in a central London exhibition, and sold in most charity shops in the UK. The copyright had been purchased, and instead of receiving £150.00 he chose to have a music centre.

David's progress was immense. He'd begun to acquire Certificates in Education. The funding office, though, were never informed of David's progress. He'd now been at this hospital for four years – two years longer than he should have been. The fees had now increased to £500 per day. David now had another consultant psychiatrist, who was attached to the hospital bungalows, and a different hospital social worker.

4. BETRAYAL OF MINDS

David had suffered problems with asthma, persistent tachycardia, problems with his back and problems with his nose. For all of these conditions, I relentlessly requested that he be examined by a doctor, but this, of course, didn't happen.

The hospital social worker said that she'd visit me at home to discuss David moving on to a further new establishment. When she called, she said that she needed my support to secure funding for a place to be kept there for David. I said I would help if I could. Although I hadn't yet seen this new establishment, I wrote a letter to their funding office in support of their funding David. I believed I was doing the right thing − I believed it would become easier for me to secure David's ultimate freedom at some stage.

The hospital social worker said that David was a young man and needed his independence. David's psychiatrist and hospital social worker asked me if I would like to go and see this establishment. I told them I'd take a look at the place as soon as I could. A few weeks passed, and finally, after much pressure from both the hospital social worker, David's psychiatrist and the administrator of the new establishment, I went to visit it. After travelling for nearly three hours by car, we finally arrived. There was scaffolding erected at the front and side entrances, accompanied by sandbags and builder's gravel. I went into the reception area, where I was greeted by an administration assistant. She took me into a sitting room, where she began asking me questions about David. The only trouble was that there was no privacy. I found myself discussing David in front of other patients. I was given tea in a dirty cup, which I fully admit to emptying into a most conveniently-placed potted plant. We were now shown the rest of the building. I came across lots of rooms which were clearly unfinished. The one chosen for David was damp and smelled of rotting cabbages, which I remarked about.

The grounds were a mess; there was a rather large cow grazing nearby. The nearest town was some two hours' drive away, and I believed that David would be very lonely here. The railway station was in the middle of nowhere and it was surrounded by forest. I was told that David would be given a mobile phone and that he could go out to the pub, which was also two hours' drive away. I was also told that if he had a girlfriend, he couldn't take her back to the establishment. They showed me a caravan-type shed within the grounds. I walked inside a tiny area and was told this was where the arts and craft classes were held. I wasn't impressed. Although the place wasn't up to scratch, I thought if this is what David wanted, then I wouldn't stand in his way. It wasn't until the administrator of this establishment informed me, whilst walking through the grounds, that David's psychiatrist was a personal friend of the owner of this establishment, that I felt things weren't right. I asked the administrator how much the fees were at this place, and she told me they were £1,200 per week. When I got home, I phoned David. I asked him if he'd seen the establishment. He said he had. I asked him if he'd rather come home to me.

He said 'Yes, Mum, I would, but they've told me I can't.'

'Never mind what they've said, I'm telling you, you can come home.'

David seemed very pleased at hearing this. However, the hospital social worker and the psychiatrist informed David that he couldn't return home to me. At the same time, they told me that David wished to be placed at this new establishment and didn't want to come home.

I received a letter from the local social services office, saying they'd like to visit me. I wrote a letter back, saying that over the past six years since David had been in hospital, not one of the social workers had bothered to see whether I was dead or alive. Suddenly now they wished to see me. I'd had reason to complain in the past about the social worker who was coming. This lady had once turned up for a hospital Mental Health Review meeting. She'd said at that meeting that she felt David should remain in hospital. Realising that perhaps she hadn't done her homework and was merely going on old notes, I challenged her views on the grounds that she really wasn't qualified to give her opinion when she'd never met David. She'd never even met me, and only met David for the first time at this meeting. I felt very strongly, based on this – her views shouldn't be accepted. They were accepted merely because everyone concerned wanted David to go to the new establishment.

They wanted him to remain in hospital until funding had been agreed, and it appeared they didn't mind what they said or wrote in order for this to be achieved. David had been attending further education classes whilst at the bungalow and had received certificates of achievements – but the funding office knew nothing of these achievements. If they'd known, they would have withdrawn funding immediately. After all, David's care had been funded for the past six years out of the pockets of taxpayers, including myself. This hospital, along with Social Services, had succeeded in deceiving the funding office, in order to procure further funding. I remembered quite clearly the period of time set by the funding office was only two years.

We picked David up from the hospital, and on the way home David told us about how he'd become attached to one of the female nursing staff called Esther. He also told us how deeply upset he'd become with a new nursing assistant, called Peter. David had told Peter how he liked Esther.

Peter, turned to David and said: 'She's not for the likes of you, so get your F........ mind off it.'

I decided to raise a complaint at his remark, which I felt was uncalled for and unprofessional. Especially as staff are not allowed to have any kind of relationship with patients. This is widely known and respected. But I felt that it didn't hurt to dream of normality in one's life, and that is all David had done. Why, then, should a person who is supposed to understand the mentally ill destroy this dream, and be so rude, too? My complaint had the desired affect −Peter, was transferred! When you've been around mentally ill people as much as I have, you can tell at first glance if someone has experienced mental health problems. Likewise, I can also tell if a nursing assistant is genuine or not − it's a kind of intuitive feeling, which I believe anyone can have. After all the first four years experiences, when David became ill where nursing staff were concerned, I'd learned the difference between dedication and the lack of it.

On one of David's visits home, I took him shopping. I've always supported charity shops, and although David wasn't keen, I went into the local charity shop - Scope Charity shop in the Town Centre of Hatfield

David became interested in some old CDs and decided to buy one. A woman whom I'd known for a few years namely Bridget, came up to me and asked: 'How's your son?'

David was busy looking at yet more CDs at the other end of the shop.

I replied: 'Four steps forward and one back.'

She then said: 'Have you heard of euthanasia?'

I said nothing.

She went on to say: 'Because when you're not around any more to look after him, he'll become a burden to the state and to taxpayers like myself.'

David, by this time, was standing behind me. He'd heard what she'd said, and he too said nothing. We were both lost for words. David left the CDs he was going to buy on the counter and we both walked out of the shop.

He then said to me: 'I'm so glad I'm not her son, Mum.'

I began walking home with David, becoming more and more angry with every step I took. What planet had this woman been living on over the past few years?

Was she not aware of where she worked? Did she not know what this charity was for? When I got home, I immediately put pen to paper and

Josephine Brown

wrote this poem:

BUT STILL I RISE
You may malign, you may judge
What price to pay for ultimate love –
The love a mother has for her son.
A mental illness which has now begun
To be met with such prejudice and
Beguiled disguise –

But, Still I Rise.

To await hope where none is to hand,
To be met with the closing of doors
One after another.
Feelings of inferiority, as to many I'm just
An unfortunate mother.
The tears are there, but I do not cry –

But, Still I Rise.

Hopes and dreams of a mother become
shattered by others.
 To have been blessed with a courageous
Young man. The doors remain bolted and tied,
One day to burst open wide, awaiting this
Child to fly –

But, Still I Rise.

Cruel words I endure and receive
Inner feelings I neither deny nor believe
That the mentally ill will one day, not
Be perceived as evil and vile.
The arrival of arrogance, mischief and lies

BETRAYAL OF MINDS

Yesterday, today and tomorrow
A heart that is filled only with compassionate pride
I remain hopeful, yet fearful, of the future years
Expecting only heartache, ridicule and
An abundance of tears −

But, Still I Rise.

I wrote to Scope's head office and raised my concerns regarding their shop assistant's remarks. I received an apology.   This apology, however, meant nothing to me or to David, as this shop assistant still works in the shop. Both David and myself feel that we cannot walk into the shop whilst she remains.

When David had to return to the hospital, he displayed much self-control, for which he gained my admiration, and which he will always have. He never complained, and yet, as we drew nearer to the hospital, I could feel him becoming tense and apprehensive.

Later, I received a phone call from him, saying that he'd been hit across the head with a frying pan. He'd been cooking, and another patient was fed up with David muttering to himself and asked him to shut up. David didn't hear him and the patient hit him. I said to David, who hadn't been seriously hurt, that perhaps it would be better if he kept quiet when cooking.

David replied: 'I have to keep reminding myself

constantly of what comes next.'

I said: 'Like what?'

'Well, I have to think, if I'm doing chips, whether I should take my potatoes out the freezer.'

'Why do you put potatoes in the freezer, David?' I asked.

'Well, they'll go off if I don't, won't they?'

Why, I thought, hadn't a member of staff informed David that you don't usually put potatoes in the freezer?

David was at a hospital charging £500.00 per day. He was supposed to be learning skills to enable him to become independent. Yet, no-one had told David a few basics in storing food. I decided to give David a few cookery lessons when he next came home, so, at the very least, he'd never be hit across the head again by anyone's frying pan.

David did mutter to himself a lot and this could become irritating, but you don't go through what David has and come out totally unscathed.

David could only be given 500 mg per day of his medication, because he suffered persistent tachycardia. He should have more, but this would be dangerous. He also suffers with asthma, along with the injuries he's received in hospital that have never been treated.

His nose, for instance, has taken a beating, and I believed it to have been broken at some stage, because David has difficulty breathing through his nose. I've also been informed that should he suffer an epileptic fit due to his medication, his heart would not withstand it, and his life could very well cease.

This information only made me more determined to secure his freedom. I'd only known my son for just 13 years before all hell had let loose, and I wanted to spend time with him, however short that time may be.

It had become apparent that we had now entered a war between us, Social Services, David's psychiatrist, one of David's solicitors and, of course, the new establishment, who were ready, indeed only too willing, and anxious to have David as one of their clients. After all, the taxpayers again would be funding the venture to the tune, as previously mentioned, of £1,200.00 per week, and rising. Throughout David's illness there were two songs I'd kept playing whilst on my way to visiting him. The first track was by Aretha Franklin – 'I had a Dream' and the second was by R Kelly – 'I believe I can Fly'. In these two songs, I found the strength to believe in myself and the decisions I was making. After all, there were people from all walks of life who'd given up on their children after discovering they'd been diagnosed with schizophrenia. There was also many who'd stuck by their children, only to feel a great loss in their lives, hopelessness followed by isolation, with the added burden of stigmatisation.

5. A BATTLE TO BE FOUGHT

I believed beyond a shadow of doubt that David no longer wanted to go to the new establishment. I no longer believed what David's hospital social worker, the local social workers and also his psychiatrist were saying – that David didn't want to come home. At the same time, they were all telling David that he couldn't go home. It was time, I felt, to contact a friend in the funding office, whom I'd known for many years. I never kept in regular contact, but hoped she still worked in the same office. I phoned this lady, who confirmed that David was only supposed to be at the second hospital for a maximum period of two years. She'd never been informed of David's achievements whilst he was at the hospital, nor of any progress he had made. Had she known, she would have withdrawn funding immediately and without hesitation. I explained to her that David wished to come home and I wanted him home. I informed her that I'd instructed a solicitor on his behalf and I'd also been able to obtain a solicitor for myself. I explained to her my mistrust of the local Social Services department, David's hospital social worker and his psychiatrist. It also came to my attention a few weeks later that, if David needed treatment in the new establishment, the call-out fee would be over £500.00. This would be payable to David's current psychiatrist, as there was no RMO (Resident Mental Health Officer) at the new establishment. Such fees are, I feel, exorbitant and unnecessary.

An application had been made for a Mental Health Review Tribunal; it was to take place on the 14th August 2003. Knowing that we were outnumbered, we enlisted the support of my brother-in-law, Mr John Burrow, whose efforts were amazing, considering he was in his early 70s. John has a very wide understanding of mental health matters, and at one time presided at meetings.

We were similar to the Three Musketeers – we didn't, of course, carry weapons, but you could say our weapons were strategies that even Winston Churchill would have been proud of! My legal representation was performed by a panel representative, a young woman called Natasha.

David's solicitor - Deborah, came recommended by Natasha. I specifically requested that both solicitors liaise with each other, but this didn't happen. Natasha, had been promised that she would see documentation relating to David via Deborah, before the Tribunal date. The day before the Hearing, however, no papers were forthcoming, and Deborah, it seemed had disappeared from the planet. Meanwhile, I was sent letters suggesting that I meet with the local Social Services team, who'd still not met either David or myself. I sent them a letter saying that due to the fact they'd not bothered to see me or David in the past, I felt it was too late for them to be now showing an interest. They wrote back to me, suggesting that David should, indeed, go to the new establishment.   I informed them that David wouldn't be going to any further establishments, as David would be coming home. David's hospital social worker was also busy persuading David that he must go to the new establishment. So David was now having a lot of pressure put on him by all sides, which was wrong. It was, after all, David's application, and I was going to see that it remained David's application.   An easy enough task, you may think, but not so. David's own solicitor - Deborah, was suggesting to him that he should go to the new establishment, but David was having none of it.   He instructed her that he wished to come home. I spoke to Natasha, and requested her to write to Deborah, telling her of her client's instructions – that he wished to be discharged home, and to cease telling her client that he must go to the new establishment.

 On the day of the Hearing, Mike and I picked John up and we travelled to the hospital. We'd arrived one hour early so that we could spend some time with David.   We approached the bungalow and asked to see David.   Deborah, came out to us and told us that she wished to go over the papers with David. I told her that I wished to see my son.

She replied: 'Can you come back in half an hour?'

I agreed, but our attempts to see David before the

Hearing were in vain. Ten minutes before the actual Hearing, David came running up to me, saying that he no longer wished to see his solicitor, let alone have her represent him.

He told us that he'd been smoking a cigarette and she'd asked him not to smoke – saying that he had to behave correctly in front of the Tribunal. She'd also tried to get him to agree to going to the new establishment. David said she was like an old granny – telling him what to do and how to behave. But David's experience of Tribunal Hearings was immense. He knew how to behave and he also knew that he'd not be able to smoke inside. He never, of course, thought that he'd be instructed to put his cigarette out, or become bullied <u>before</u> the Hearing. Deborah, walked through to a back room – presumably where she'd been met by David's psychiatrist and Social Services. The meeting would now begin.

The Hearing was delayed by about two hours. David was getting agitated, and Mike, John and myself weren't far behind. We were, in fact, becoming quite cross. The judge who had agreed to hear David's Application had been presiding on a previous case for the Home Office. However, David had never been the subject of a Home Office issue. The Clerk to the Tribunal came over to us and apologised for the delay, and we went into the Hearing.All the Social workers, both the local team and hospital Social Worker who'd been connected to both David and myself - had not submitted their reports to the panel, despite having been given some three months' prior notice. The judge wasn't at all happy with this. It further transpired that Deborah had all the relevant documentation on the day of the hearing, but no one else did! It meant that David's Hearing would now have to be adjourned for a further three months. The Judge told Social Services, basically, that they needed to get their act together. After the Judge had Adjourned the Hearing, Deborah piped up with her 'proposals' for David. The judge had to remind her again that the case had now been adjourned. On the way out, I spoke to the Judge and told him that I needed to get David out of Kneesworth Hospital, because his medical issues weren't being addressed.

I thanked him for his help and we shook hands. David went back to the bungalow with Mike and John, whilst Natasha and I went to the hospital restaurant. We asked John and Mike to join us there. We'd often had a meal on other occasions at the restaurant. I asked the receptionist if it would be OK to have a meal. She said it would be fine. We chose our meal and sat down. A Clerk to the Tribunal was also having a meal. Within a few minutes, David's hospital social worker- Gill, requested that Natasha and I leave immediately. She informed us that we were not allowed to be in the restaurant.

I said to her: 'Yes, OK, but can you go away now,

please?'

 We began eating our meal, but Gill came over to us yet again and requested us to leave.

This time, Natasha said to her: 'When we've finished our meal, we will leave. Now please go away.'

Meanwhile, Mike and John had tried to enter the restaurant, but were met by Gill, David's hospital social worker. She informed them they were not allowed into the restaurant. She took them into a room and said she'd get them a sandwich. Mike and John were not impressed. Natasha and I finished our meal in our own time and left the restaurant. We managed to find Mike and John.

We were then met by Deborah.

She looked at her diary and said: 'I can only get to see David possibly the week after next because I'm at Broadmoor on Tuesday and again on Wednesday, Thursday and Friday.'

 I looked into my folder and said: 'Well, I can't make it either, 'cos I'm at Woolworths on Wednesday, John Lewis's on Thursday and Marks & Sparks on Friday.' I knew that Deborah would never represent my son ever again.   I also knew David was absolutely terrified of her, and also she appeared to be sitting on both sides of the fence.

BETRAYAL OF MINDS

She was ignoring David's instructions (that he just wanted to come home)She was also applying pressure on David to go to the new establishment and totally ignoring his repeated instructions - that he just wanted to go home. On the other hand, David liked my representative, Natasha. She was a very dedicated caring person, and this she had displayed. She agreed to act for David. I decided to seek another firm of solicitors to represent me. I wanted David to have someone whom he felt comfortable with and whom I knew wouldn't terrify him. So I wrote a letter to Deborah's firm of Solicitors, on behalf of David, saying that Deborah's services would no longer be required and that I would be raising a complaint to the Law Society about her conduct towards David.

Despite David having signed a 'Consent to Act' form for Natasha to now represent him, this was ignored by Deborah's firm of solicitors. They refused to send the papers to Natasha's firm of solicitors. . They objected to David choosing my representative, Natasha. I raised a complaint about Deborah's firm of solicitors to the Law Society.

My complaint raised two issues − firstly, that their solicitor - Deborah, had refused to take instructions from her client, stating that he wished to return home to his family. Secondly, that this firm of solicitors had failed to submit David's file to

David's chosen representative, Natasha.

This complaint had been registered and I was invited to voice my issues before a Complaints Board. But I discovered that one of the partners of Deborah's firm sat on the panel. So I didn't pursue my complaints, as I felt our case could be compromised. It may not have been the case, but I simply didn't feel comfortable. Did I feel bruised and battered emotionally? Yes, I did. This only made me more determined than ever to continue to fight to have my son home.

I telephoned the establishment in Norfolk and said: 'You can give the bed you're saving for David to someone else, as my son will not be going to your establishment.'

However, they said that they believed he would. But Natasha was unable to represent David now − Deborah's firm of Solicitors, had, it would seem, become vengeful. Instead, I enlisted the help of a Mr Ian Campbell to bring about a Nearest Relatives Application, and he, in turn, recommended a lady Solicitor called Sarah Burke to represent David.

I'd been informed the new Hearing would be on the 20th October 2003.

David's hospital social worker Gill, and the local social worker, Angela, had succeeded in obstructing David's Hearing by delaying his

BETRAYAL OF MINDS

Application – they hadn't submitted the necessary paperwork on the 14th August 2003.

It also came to my attention that these individuals requested the funding office to obtain funding for David to attend the new establishment, just a few days after they'd managed to delay David's Hearing. Their request had been refused on the grounds that I'd informed the funding office not only of David's achievements whilst at Kneesworth, but also had stated I wished my son to be discharged home, and that, more importantly, David wanted to come home. It also came to light that Social Services were looking towards obtaining a Guardianship Order. This would have diminished any rights I may have had over David's future care.

I wrote to the Mental Health Review Panel, giving them step-by-step information as to what was happening. I further requested that copies of my letters be sent to the Judge whom I'd met briefly at the previous Adjourned Hearing, for his interest only. I was invited to attend a meeting at the hospital with David's hospital social worker Gill and the local Social Worker - Angela. They did their very best to try to get me to change my mind. I informed them that I categorically wanted my son to come home.

David, who also attended this meeting, voiced the same request.   Meanwhile, my Solicitor, Ian, called at my home one evening. He'd come to see David, who was home on a visit. He gave us a copy of a Report that had been written by David's hospital social worker Gill and David's psychiatrist. It had been this document that Natasha, had tried to obtain from Deborah, but hadn't been able to. This Report however, had to be requested by my Solicitor Ian, before the Judge whilst attending David's disastrous Application. This Report had written on the front cover in large bold letters 'Not For Disclosure to Patient or Family'. It further went on to say: 'This document contains information regarding the patient's relationship with his mother. We believe this information would adversely affect the health and welfare of the patient if it were shown to his mother'.

On reading the contents of this report, I was amazed. No wonder they'd not wished me to have sight of it. I will mention only a few remarks in this report:

First, the psychiatrist remarked that David had never fitted in with his peer group and had no friends when he was 13. This was untrue. Had she simply asked David about his friends, including girlfriends at this time, he could have supplied her with a list.

She also stated that David was 'a danger to himself and to others'. If, indeed, this was correct, why had she remained silent, knowing that David had, for the past two years, been allowed to go out unaccompanied, to go shopping, and to visit the library, the local pub and the video shop? He travelled by public transport or simply walked – the town was about one mile away from the hospital. Would it not have been her duty to have stopped all David's trips out if she really believed he was a danger to himself and to others?

I believed, along with my Solicitor Ian, that this report would not be upheld in a Court of Law, due to the fact it was an absolute contradiction of terms. In order for David to go out by himself, the psychiatrist herself would have had to sign the hospital's own -Special Leave 'Section 17'.

The report also mentioned that David did not like tidying up or cooking for himself. Were they not aware that most young men don't like doing household chores? I wondered if family life was that alien to them.

I decided that I would respond to their report by submitting a report of my own. In this report, I commented how the hospital social worker Gill, and David's psychiatrist's report had rigidly followed the text books, and that, it seemed, they had little or no understanding of the illness from which David suffered. This was pretty scary, considering these people are dealing with people's lives. In this case, they were denying an individual his freedom. Not very impressive when you think that the fees were some £500.00 per day, and rising. Neither of these individuals knew my son very well at all, despite having spent long periods of time with him.

I sent a copy of the original report to the Mental Health Review Panel. Had it gone unchallenged, it could have kept David in hospital for a very long time. Reports of any kind should be seen by all of the parties involved in the case. They must either be agreed upon or, as in David's case, challenged. After all, such reports can be very damaging, if found to be incorrect. Especially if a patient has to remain for many years in hospital or another establishment, never knowing why.

It is my opinion that an independent office (not attached to any particular hospital) should be set up in order to automatically challenge or question the continued detainment of any mentally ill or physically disabled person. (Similar to that of a Scrutiny Panel) This would also ensure, that patients who are truly dangerous are not set free. This would cut costs dramatically to the taxpayers, but, more importantly, the Mental Health Service providers would be investigated more vigorously. This, in turn, would cut the workload created and save the Mental Health Review Panel from attending Tribunal Hearings without having the necessary documentation. Such documentation would have to be provided by the independent office to the Panel. This would avoid unnecessary delays orchestrated by social workers, as in the case of David's first application, where the obstruction it caused led to an immeasurable amount of stress for all concerned. The persons in this independent office should be changed periodically or moved about from one district to another, in order to avoid personal feelings or views becoming an issue for any particular patient whom they may have seen.

Consultant psychiatrists should not be allowed to organise the release of any particular patient without first having had at least 5 years' minimum experience in dealing with the mentally ill. Before any release of a patient, two psychiatrists (who are not known to each other) should arrive at the same decision in regard to the patient. Then, of course, the final stage would be for the independent office to agree with the decision that both consultant psychiatrists have made.

This may sound long and exhaustive, but many wrong decisions have been made in the past – sometimes, patients who should remain in hospital have been, wrongly, allowed to go back into society, with disastrous results.

Patients such as David, who should have been discharged within two years, have been, and still are, kept detained for no apparent reason other than to procure monies from the NHS, which fully admits to always being short of funds.

6. THE TRIBUNAL HEARING

On the 20th October 2003, Mike, myself and John attended the hospital for another Tribunal Hearing. David had been brought over to see us by a nursing assistant. David smiled at Sarah, his solicitor – at last he, although nervous, seemed happy, and hopeful that he'd be discharged. It's something we were all hoping for. But I couldn't dare to imagine walking out of the hospital with David, never to return.

The Hearing was on time. We entered the room – the Panel sat on one side behind a desk, along with three others. These were a psychiatrist for the Tribunal, a solicitor and a lay person. David's psychiatrist sat opposite to them. The other side consisted of Mike, myself, John, David, the hospital social worker Gill, the local social worker Angela. My solicitor, Ian, and, of course, David's solicitor, Sarah.   There was also another Social Worker called Maggie, I believe from the local Outreach Team of Social Services.

The psychiatrist for the Tribunal began firing questions at David's psychiatrist, who apologised for having a cold.   He said he'd read her comments saying that David should remain in hospital and then be placed at a new establishment, as he was a danger to himself and to others.   I've heard these words before, I thought.

BETRAYAL OF MINDS

He then asked her, if this really was her view, why had she allowed David to have unaccompanied visits home. She had also allowed him to go on holiday with his family, go to the pub, and so on. She didn't answer him − the Tribunal solicitor asked her to reply.

What could she say? I don't recall hearing her response. At this stage, Mike's chair broke and he shot forward, trying to avoid crashing to the floor.

Then, the Tribunal solicitor asked her if there had been eight assaults upon David whilst he was a patient.

She replied: 'Yes, there have been eight assaults.'

He then asked her if David had been aggressive whilst at the hospital, or refused his medication.

She replied: 'No, he's never been aggressive or refused his medication.'

They all, in turn, fired questions at each other. Now it was David's turn.

The Tribunal solicitor asked David: 'What benefit do you think you have got by being here at the hospital?'

David replied: 'I get £15.00 a week benefit.'

This reply wasn't what the solicitor had meant, but he saw the funny side of David's remark, as did we all, so there was laughter all round. Now it was my turn. The Tribunal solicitor asked me how long I'd been in denial of David's illness.

I replied: 'It took me a year to come to terms with it initially.'

I also said, without being asked, that I knew the warning signs of his illness and, if I was concerned about David's mental state, I would notify the mental health services.

It was decided by all members of the Tribunal that David be discharged home to me, to the absolute horror of David's psychiatrist and Social Services, but that his discharge would occur three weeks later, on Monday 17th November at 12 noon, so that arrangements could be made for David's care.

'Nice one,' I said quietly in Mike's ear.

I felt like going into the nearest pub. I didn't know whether it was safe or not to be happy. I could see the hospital staff were shocked − they couldn't believe it either. It was one of the happiest days of my life. I'd spent ten years going to see David and standing in defence of him, and now I could walk out of that hospital with David, never to return. I'd written precisely 101 letters to the

BETRAYAL OF MINDS

Mental Health Tribunal, and it had now, finally, paid off.

The 17th November 2003 arrived, and Mike and I went to collect David from the hospital. He'd said his goodbyes and the staff told me how they'd miss him, and how glad they were that David had been discharged. They also asked how we'd managed to accomplish it.

I didn't wish to seem unsociable, but I really didn't want to stand and chat. Both David and I couldn't wait to get out of the place. On the way home, David told me that he'd experienced problems walking. He said his leg was really hurting him. I asked him if he'd had an accident – he said he hadn't. Mike has never speeded whilst driving, but we simply couldn't get away from the hospital fast enough. I remember that 'Land of Hope and Glory' was playing on the radio. How appropriate, I thought, as today we too had won a battle. A battle that had turned our lives upside down and inside out, and that had unnecessarily cost David ten years of his life.

We arrived home, but after a few days, David still couldn't believe his luck. He kept asking when he would have to return.

A meeting was arranged with Social Services, as they now had a Duty of Care towards David. There are social workers who do a good job, and for this I'm thankful, as I'm sure the rest of the population are. However, the only local social worker I've really liked was a woman called Maggie − what an absolute gem she was.

But it must be said that there are also some social workers who are 'rotten apples', such as Angela, who visited us later. We looked at each other with absolute horror − we simply couldn't stand each other's company, for obvious reasons. I'd raised a complaint about both the hospital social worker Gill, and Angela, whose actions had deliberately delayed David's original Hearing on the 14th August 2003, as they hadn't submitted their documentation. So there was, of course, no love lost between us. Unfortunately, David, now free, had to attend yet another meeting with the local team of Social Services, and, of course, guess who lay in wait…..

Before the meeting began, we were shown into a room where, to my surprise, David's hospital psychiatrist at Kneesworth was sitting, looking rather miserable, I thought. Next to her was David's initial psychiatrist from the QE11 Hospital in Welwyn Garden City. The psychiatrist who'd initially sent David to Kneesworth hospital in Cambridge without my prior knowledge. Social Services were also present, but not the hospital social worker Gill, of course.

I entered the room feeling as if I had just won a fight, but, of course, there were no cheers of delight from my awaiting audience. My solicitor, Ian, sat next to me, and David's solicitor, Sarah, sat next to him. Mike and John also sat with us. My day of judgment had now arrived – what had they all got to say for themselves? This will be most interesting, I thought, wearing one of my most wicked smiles.

Furthermore, I was thinking to myself: 'My son's out of your clutches now – what the bloody hell are you going to do about it?'

To my amazement, David's, psychiatrist from Kneesworth House Hospital said to his original psychiatrist: from the QE11 Hospital in Hertfordshire. 'Should David become unwell in the future, he must be allowed to bypass the local Accident and Emergency procedures – his bed will be waiting for him at her hospital.'

She further said she didn't expect David to last longer than two months at home with me.

Ian, my solicitor, just looked at her and said: 'Oh, really'.

David's hospital psychiatrist from Kneesworth House Hospital then looked angrily at Ian and said to him: 'I'm not talking to you'.

Ian and Sarah had been absolutely brilliant – their help in obtaining David's freedom had been worthy of an award, if not in this life then, surely, in the next. Their support had been invaluable and I'd have no hesitation in instructing them again.

At that meeting, everyone agreed to help David and myself, but we knew we wouldn't need their help. After all, we'd achieved the impossible. We'd fought a battle. We had, I believe, sent a firm message to all concerned that we'd never again tolerate such abuse of our rights by financially motivated individuals, no matter how many letters they may have after their names. If a mentally ill patient, who was initially described, by David's Psychiatrist, as being "a danger to himself and to others" , was actually so, then the Mental Health Review Tribunal are more than qualified, to work it out for themselves. (Although its certainly worthwhile keeping them fully informed as to developments) My defence and utter defiance, along with the help of Mike, John, Ian and Sarah, had brought an end to what I can only describe as a ten year nightmare of events. David had never killed anyone. He'd simply suffered, at a very early age a serious mental illness. For this, he'd lost 10 years of his life. I do not deny that David needed to become hospitalised, but feel very strongly his illness, should have been successfully treated within a maximum period of just 3 years.

Would David and I now find peace? No, it would seem this wasn't going to happen – not just yet, at any rate. David had been completely traumatised by having been detained for all of his teenage years, and he simply couldn't believe he was now free.   If an ambulance drove past, David immediately presumed it was for him. Every day he remained at home, he showed signs of his insecurity.   We gave him support and understanding at these times, although we couldn't simply wipe out the last ten years. We can make David's time with us less traumatic, and give him hope that he can and will achieve his goals in life, even if such goals and achievements take longer than he'd expected.

David often comments about the day I visited him at the hospital bungalow shortly after having survived a stroke. The staff knew I was ill. I was just about to return home when a member of staff said goodbye to me. From her tone, she sounded as though she was happy to see me leave. I couldn't blame her for having that thought, but I went up to her and said: 'Even if I die tomorrow, please don't feel you can relax. Because I'll be able to see you, but you won't be able to see me!'

She didn't reply, neither did I expect her to, but I believe my words had hit home, because the very next day she allowed David to go to the pub on the day before my next visit. In fact, he'd already been to the pub! She also insisted that he phone me to see how I was.

7. LACK OF GP CARE

Over the past weeks, David had been limping. We also needed to get his injuries he'd received whilst at Kneesworth hospital checked out. I made an appointment to see his GP. This GP had known David since the onset of his illness in 1993/94. I, therefore, was expecting some kind of understanding from this man.

We arrived at the surgery and explained to the GP that David had been experiencing a problem with his leg. We also explained that David had suffered a problem with his nose and eyes. To my horror, this doctor suggested that David's apparent physical medical problems be referred to his psychiatrist!

If I went to a GP and was suffering leg, eye and nose problems, I'd be somewhat alarmed if my GP said that my ailments needed to be sorted out by a psychiatrist!

'Where's this man coming from?' I thought.

He never examined David, nor did he treat him, except to give him a prescription for paracetamol.

However, the GP said to David: 'I don't know whether these tablets are compatible with your other medication.'

BETRAYAL OF MINDS

Could he have not looked it up in one of his medical books? After all, if these prescribed tablets did have an adverse affect on David, it could send him back to hospital again, the very place we were trying to avoid.

This visit had become a complete waste of time. We left the surgery with David still limping along the road. I felt so angry and, again, so very sorry for David. I told him that I'd make an appointment to see my GP, who was at a completely different surgery. In fact, I told him that I'd register him with my GP so that he would never have to put up with the apparent lack of care he'd received at his own GP's practice. I duly saw the practice receptionist and completed the forms for David, and also for Mike, who'd agreed that the first GP (who was also Mike's GP) had acted deplorably towards David. My GP practice had seen and treated my daughter, Jane, successfully, earlier in the year, and she hadn't been one of their patients, so I believed my GP would be better than the last doctor. So pleased had I been in the past with my surgery that at Christmas, I made sure they all received a gift from me.

On Friday 26th November 2003, I telephoned my surgery to enquire as to whether both David and Mike would be able to register with my GP. After speaking to the receptionist I spoke to my GP's secretary, who suggested that I collect the registration forms. I completed these, told her that my son suffered with mental health problems, and made an appointment for David to see my GP on 27th November.

When the time of the appointment came, David and I proceeded into my GP's room, but we were requested by her to wait outside, as she said she needed to update David's records on her computer.

We returned to the reception area and waited a further ten minutes, during which two other people went into her room. This suggested to me that my GP couldn't have been updating her computer.

The receptionist came up to us and said: 'Who said he was to come to our surgery?'

I replied: 'Social Services.'

The receptionist then disappeared.

After a further five minutes, the practice manager came up to us and said: 'We have a deal with David's surgery – they don't take our patients and we don't take theirs.'

He also suggested, whilst marching us to the front entrance, that we try a surgery nearby which, he said, takes anyone. We were never given the opportunity of seeing my GP – yet again, David had been denied treatment.   I returned to this surgery a few days later and collected Mike's registration form. It appeared this surgery were prepared to accept Mike, but not David. I thought that at least one of the GPs would have treated David, as they had, some months before, treated Jane.

David remained in pain for the next few days. I believe my GP had discriminated against David due to his mental health problems, and I consequently registered complaints to both the General Medical Council and The Complaints Department of the NHS, regarding both David's and my GPs. The General Medical Council took a considerable time to decide on both matters. There is also another point I raised − a certain GP was employed on a part time basis at both David's and my surgeries. I pointed out that if a GP could work for both surgeries, why couldn't patients move from one to the other?

I received a letter from the General Medical Council saying that they'd had a word with both surgeries, and that David's GP had acted correctly. I think most people would be very alarmed if they went to see their GP suffering from a painful leg and their GP referred them to a psychiatrist! I was absolutely appalled and disgusted at their findings. If GPs do not treat the mentally ill for whatever reason, does this not pose a potential risk to the general public? If a mentally ill person seeks advice and is refused it by a doctor, then any offence this person later commits may be seen as the doctor's fault, resulting from the failure to treat him or her in the first instance. Any liability for such an offence should be the GP's.

Sadly, the age-old stigma of mental illness is seen again. These two GP Practices, displaying signs at their Surgeries which clearly stated ' We do not discriminate against age, gender, colour or disability. Had indeed, discriminated against David.

I could have understood their view not to treat David, had he been aggressive or dirty and smelly. But David was clean and non-aggressive. He remained very polite throughout this ordeal, despite his obvious pain.

I managed to register on the list that 'takes anyone', and David was eventually treated for his painful leg.

However, the GPs at this surgery were friends of David's previous GP. I required treatment for my back, but I was told by a GP that I didn't need treatment. Later, I made an appointment with a different GP, giving a false name. On that occasion, I was informed that I most certainly did require treatment for my back. Since this episode, I've been diagnosed with osteoporosis of the cervical spine, which had gone untreated from the time I initially required help from my GP, and was denied it. The time lapse had been three years. Some GPs should come with a Government Health Warning – 'If you dare criticise your GP, your health could be seriously affected'.

All NHS Complaint Trusts should become a thing of the past, as these Trusts can become biased towards those being complained against. Again, independent legal and lay persons should decide upon such complaints. We do have ombudsmen, but it is widely felt this office can also become biased. Finally, the General Medical Council has always been recognised as a body of people who can become biased against the complainant unless, of course, your case has already been proved by a solicitor, or your complaint is in regards of a death solely caused, and proved to have been caused, by a negligent doctor. The General Medical Council can take as long as one year to give a decision. This procedure is costly and outdated. When a decision has finally arrived, it's been my experience they can be wrong. Justice isn't being done for ordinary people. No-one questions these establishments, but they should do. It's time these age-old relics of society should be updated or, at the very least, become a question of parliamentary debate. It has become clear to me that changes are urgently needed to be made.

I'd been informed that if David was to suffer a full epileptic fit his life could cease. David's heart would not function under such stress. Who would treat my son, who would help me? If it has been so immensely difficult for a simple examination to be done by his GP to relieve David's physical suffering, then I can only pray that we are not put in such dire circumstances. In reality however, the continued use of clozapine could very likely cause David to suffer such a fit. We live with this possibility every day, as do thousands of other people.

David now has a team of social workers whom, I'm pleased to say, have been great. The staff at the hospital where David was first admitted are no longer working on that ward.

However, they have all been given 'promotions' within the Mental Health Services.

Schizophrenia is a serious mental illness, but it's a lot less complicated if you can separate the patient's character from the illness.

If, after reading this book, you feel your freedom is worth fighting for, then go for it, and never give up. I didn't, and I won!

Three years later – David now attends college and is studying for his GCSEs in Maths and English. He has a few friends, but the one quality I admire most in David is that he never criticises anyone, even if their comments are not what he wants to hear. His illness has made him emotionally immature to some degree, because he was so very badly treated by individuals who were supposed to look after him, both in and out of hospital. He was thrown into a lions' pit at a very early age, but he has survived. Although he was half killed and had his human rights abused, he has emerged as a courageous young man, whose mother I am extremely proud to be.

Josephine Brown

HELPFUL INFORMATION

If you should ever become mentally ill and find yourself on a Section of the Mental Health Act, please DON'T DO the following :

1   DON'T instruct an Advocacy Service attached to the hospital in which you are detained – your information may be shared with your psychiatrist, social worker and anyone else who has an interest in your circumstances. Despite this, you may be informed that your details will remain confidential!

2   DON'T instruct a solicitor recommended to you by the hospital in which you are a patient. If you're unable to go out and shop around for legal representation, ask a friend to help (preferably someone not connected to your hospital). Or find a local phone book and speak to a solicitor whom you feel comfortable with. You have the right to change your solicitor at any time, provided you sign a legal aid form agreeing to their fees for any work which they may have already done on your behalf. Make sure your instructions are as clear as possible to the person who is going to represent you. Do not, under any circumstances, be persuaded to take a course of action by your representative that you do not agree with.

3   DON'T become, in any way, intimidated by the nursing staff – you have the right to complain about them. Remember that they're being paid to look after you! If you are assaulted in any way

whatsoever by a patient − again, complain. You are in hospital to become well, and not to become the victim of another persons' aggression.

4   Should you find, after attending a Tribunal Hearing, that what has been discussed is incorrect, then write, or get someone else to write, a letter to the Mental Health Review Tribunal, on your behalf.

5   If you are moved to another hospital or establishment without warning, this is wrong. You have the right to know where, when and if you are to be transferred.

6   Take your medication, but if more than one medication is offered to you at the same time, question this. The mixing of drugs is illegal, dangerous and can be fatal.

7   IF you have previously been diagnosed with ANY form of Autism or other mental disability - INSIST this is taken into account by all those who are caring for you. Some forms of Autism can and usually does create behavioural disturbances which can be misinterpreted by psychiatrists and nursing staff to being that of "aggressive behaviour" . If this goes unrecognised - you could find yourself, either being transferred to a more secure hospital or - becoming the subject of a further Section under the Mental Health Act.

COMMENTS FROM THE AUTHOR

There are many people who suffer a serious mental illness − the symptoms may go untreated for many years, and can result in suicide. There are some who suffer a mental disorder as a result of having had it passed on to them in their genes, and others who suffer as a result of taking drugs. The most popular drug, I believe, is cannabis, but it's also the most dangerous. It causes paranoia, slowly but surely, and the consequences of this are horrendous. I believe mental illness will increase to such an extent that scientific investigations will have to be performed to obtain better medication and facilities for those who become affected. Instead of being a low priority, the mentally ill will, at some stage, become first to receive funding to eliminate the rogue genes that causes such havoc in people's lives. Serious mental illnesses will become as common as flu, but take longer to control.

There is also, without a doubt, 'trafficking' of very vulnerable mentally ill persons within the medical profession. This practice is illegal, but, nevertheless, it happens. Such 'trafficking' is as common within the Mental Health Service practitioners as slavery was many years ago, when it was forced upon the black African nations by the white aristocracy.

Furthermore, nearly one million pounds per

person is being spent by the NHS on the continued detention of 'not so seriously ill' mentally ill patients. The system appears to be 'back to front', in that often GPs and psychiatrists are not working together in treating the mentally ill properly. Due to this, the mentally ill can, and frequently do, commit crimes against the public. On the other hand, the patients who <u>can</u> be treated and given medication, like David, can and do achieve a meaningful life and are no threat to anyone.

'A danger to himself, and to others' has become a moneymaking slogan for many psychiatrists and their long-term care home colleagues. I've spent some ten years meeting many seriously mentally ill people, and if I can identify who should be allowed into the community and who should not, then surely any psychiatrist worthy of his qualifications should be able to too. I fought many battles, and won!

The Legal Aid funding for people within the Mental Health System is shortly, I believe to change (for the worse). This may mean that in future people who may be detained within the system will have less recourse to the legal facilities in order to effect discharge. This will affect especially the most "hard to reach" patients and those "without a voice, outside the system", to speak out against injustice..

David became a victim of the mental health 'trafficking' system. He didn't require ten years of his life to have been taken from him. He'd simply become a good investment. I may have lost many material items throughout my battles to obtain freedom for David, but in losing, so too have I won.

BETRAYAL OF MINDS

ACKNOWLEDGEMENTS

I give special thanks to Sarah Burke, of Burke, Niaze & Co of 470/474 Holloway Road, London N7 6NN Tel: 0207 263 7887 Emergency No: 079966 482008.

Ian Campbell of   Campbell Law Solicitors, Technology House,151 Silbury Boulevard, Milton Keynes, MK9 2BE Tel: 0845 226 8118, John & Adelaide Burrow, to Ursula Wilde of the funding office,(whose help and understanding was invaluable) and to all those present on 20th Oct 2003 from the Mental Health Review Panel, all of whom helped to secure David's freedom.

.

Lightning Source UK Ltd.
Milton Keynes UK
18 February 2011
167769UK00001B/17/A